TEDBooks

The Laws of Medicine

Field Notes from an Uncertain Science

SIDDHARTHA MUKHERJEE

TED Books
Simon & Schuster

New York London Toronto Sydney New Delhi

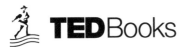

Simon & Schuster
1230 Avenue of the Americas
New York, NY 10020

Cover and interior design by: MGMT. design
Interior illustrations: *Iconographic Encyclopedia of Science, Literature, and Art*, New York: R. Garrigue, 185

Manufactured in the United States of America

10 9 8 7 6 5 4 3 2 1

Library of Congress Cataloging-in-Publication Data is available.

ISBN 978-1-4767-8484-7
ISBN 978-1-4767-8485-4 (ebook)

To Thomas Bayes (1702-1761),
who saw uncertainty with such certainty

"Are you planning to follow a career in Magical Laws, Miss Granger?" asked Scrimgeour. "No, I'm not," retorted Hermione. "I'm hoping to do some good in the world!"

J. K. Rowling

*The learned men of former ages employed a great part of
their time and thoughts searching out the hidden causes
of distemper, were curious in imagining the secret workmanship of
nature and . . . putting all these fancies together, fashioned to
themselves systems and hypotheses [that] diverted their enquiries
from the true and advantageous knowledge of things.*

John Locke

The Laws of Medicine

Years ago, as a medical student in Boston, I watched a senior surgeon operate on a woman. The surgeon, call him Dr. Castle, was a legend among the surgical residents. About six feet tall, with an imposing, formal manner that made the trainees quake in their clogs, he spoke in a slow, nasal tone that carried the distinct drawl of the South. There was something tensile in his build—more steel wire than iron girder—as if his physique had been built to illustrate the difference between stamina and strength. He began rounds at five every morning, then moved down to the operating theaters in the basement by six fifteen, and worked through the day into the early evening. He spent the weekends sailing near Scituate in a one-mast sloop that he had nicknamed *The Knife*.

The residents worshipped Castle not only for the precision of his technique, but also because of the quality of his teaching. Other surgeons may have been kinder, gentler instructors, but the key to Castle's teaching method was supreme self-confidence. He was so technically adept at surgery—so masterful at his craft—that he allowed the students to do most of the operating, knowing that he could anticipate their mistakes or correct them swiftly after. If a resident nicked an artery during an operation, a lesser surgeon might step in nervously to seal the bleeding vessel. Castle would step back and fold his arms, look quizzically at the resident, and wait for him or her to react. If the stitch came too late, Castle's hand would reach out, with the speed and precision of a falcon's talon, to pinch off the bleeding vessel, and he would stitch it himself, shaking his head, as if mumbling to himself, "Too little, too late." I have never seen senior residents in surgery, grown men and women with six or eight years of operating experience, so deflated by the swaying of a human head.

The case that morning was a woman in her fifties with a modest-size tumor in her lower intestine. We were scheduled to begin at six fifteen, as usual, but the resident assigned to the case had called in sick. A new resident was paged urgently from the wards, and he came quickly into the operating room, tugging his gloves on. Castle walked up to the CAT scans hung on the fluorescent lightbox, studied them silently for a while, then moved his head ever so slightly, signaling the first incision. There was a reverential moment as he stretched out his right hand and the nurse handed him the scalpel. The surgery began without incident.

About half an hour later, the operation was still under perfect control. Some surgeons liked to blast music in the operating room—rock and roll and Brahms were common choices—but Castle preferred silence. The resident was working fast and doing well. The only advice that Castle had offered was to increase the size of the incision to fully expose the inner abdomen. "If you can't name it, you can't cut it," he said.

But then the case took a quick turn. As the resident reached down to cut the tumor out of the body, the blood vessels surrounding it began to leak. At first, there was only a trickle, and then a few more spurts. In a few minutes about a teaspoon of blood had run into in the surgical field, obscuring the view. The carefully exposed tissues were submerged in a crimson flood. Castle stood by the side, his hands folded, watching.

The resident was clearly flustered. I watched a pool of sweat forming over his brow, mirroring the pool of blood in front of him. "Does this patient have a known bleeding disorder?" he asked, his desperation mounting. "Was she on a blood thinner?" Usually he would have studied the chart the night before and known all the answers—but he had hurriedly been assigned to the case.

"What if you didn't know?" said Castle. "What if I told you that I didn't know?" His hands had already reached into the woman's abdomen and closed the vessels shut. The patient was safe, but the resident looked devastated.

But then, it was as if a tiny bolt of knowledge had moved, like an electric arc, between Castle and his resident. The resident modified his approach. He walked over, past the surgical drapes above the woman's head, to confer with the anesthesiologist. He confirmed that the anesthesia was adequate and the patient was safely sedated. Then he returned to the surgical field and blotted out the remnant blood with some gauze. Now, he began cutting around the blood vessels when he could, charting their course with the tip of his Babcock forceps, or separating them with his fingers with exquisite delicacy, as if polishing the strings of a Stradivarius. Each time he neared a blood vessel, he turned the blade of the scalpel to its flat side and dissected with his hands, or moved farther out, leaving the vessel untouched. It took significantly longer, but there was no further bleeding. An hour later, with Castle nodding approvingly, the resident closed the incision. The tumor was out.

We walked out of the operating room in silence. "You might want to go and check her chart now," Castle said. There was a note of tenderness in his characteristic nasal twang. "It's easy to make perfect decisions with perfect information. Medicine asks you to make perfect decisions with imperfect information."

. . . .

This book is about information, imperfection, uncertainty, and the future of medicine. When I began medical school in the fall of 1995, the curriculum seemed perfectly congruent to the requirements of the discipline: I studied cell biology, anatomy, physiology, pathology, and pharmacology. By the end of the four years, I could list the five branches of the facial nerve, the chemical reactions that metabolize proteins in cells, and parts of the human body that I did not even know I possessed. I felt poised to begin practicing real medicine.

But as I advanced through my training—becoming an intern, then a resident, a fellow in oncology, and then an attending doctor treating patients with cancer—I found that a crucial piece of my education was missing. Yes, I needed the principles of cell biology to understand why, say, a platelet transfusion lasts only two weeks in most patients (platelets live in the body for only about two weeks). Anatomy helped me recall why a man had woken up from a surgical procedure with his entire lower body paralyzed (an unusual artery that supplies the lower spinal cord had become blocked by a clot, resulting in a "stroke" of the spinal cord, not the brain). An equation from pharmacology reminded me why one antibiotic was dosed four times a day while its close molecular cousin was given only once a day (the two chemicals decay at different rates in the body).

But all this information could, I soon realized, be looked up in a book or found by a single click on the Web. The information that was missing was what to *do* with information—especially when the data was imperfect, incomplete, or uncertain. Was it appropriate to treat a forty-year-old woman with acute leukemia with an aggressive bone-marrow transplant if her health was declining rapidly? At first glance, textbooks and published clinical trials gave you an answer. In this instance standard wisdom held that patients with declining health and performance should not be given a transplant. But what if that answer did not apply to *this* woman, with *this* history, in *this* particular crisis? What if the leukemia itself was causing the rapid decline? If she asked about her prognosis, I could certainly quote a survival rate pulled from a trial—but what if she was an outlier?

My medical education had taught me plenty of facts, but little about the spaces that live between facts. I could write a thesis on the physiology of vision. But I had no way to look through the fabric of confabulation spun by a man with severe lung disease who was prescribed "home oxygen," but gave a false address out of embarrassment because he had no "home." (The next morning, I got an irate phone call from the company that had attempted delivery of three canisters—to a Boston storefront that sold auto parts.)

I had never expected medicine to be such a lawless, uncertain world. I wondered if the compulsive naming of parts, diseases, and chemical reactions—frenulum, otitis, glycolysis—was a mechanism invented by doctors to defend themselves against a largely unknowable sphere of knowledge. The profusion of facts obscured a deeper and more significant problem: the reconciliation between knowledge (certain, fixed, perfect, concrete) and clinical wisdom (uncertain, fluid, imperfect, abstract).

This book began as a means for me to discover tools that might guide me through a reconciliation between these two spheres of knowledge. The "laws of medicine," as I describe them in this book, are really laws of uncertainty, imprecision, and incompleteness. They apply equally to all disciplines of knowledge where these forces come into play. They are laws of imperfection.

The stories in this book are of real people and cases, but I have changed names and identities and altered some contexts and diagnoses. The conversations were not recorded verbatim, but have been paraphrased from my memory. Some situations, tests, and trials have also been changed to maintain the anonymity of patients and doctors.

In *Harry Potter*, that philosophical treatise disguised as a children's book, a teacher of wizardry asks Hermione Granger, the young witch-in-training, whether she wishes to learn the Magical Laws to pursue a career in magic. "No," says Granger. She wishes to learn the laws so that she can do some good in the world. For Granger, magical laws do not exist to perpetuate magic. They exist as tools to interpret the world.

. . . .

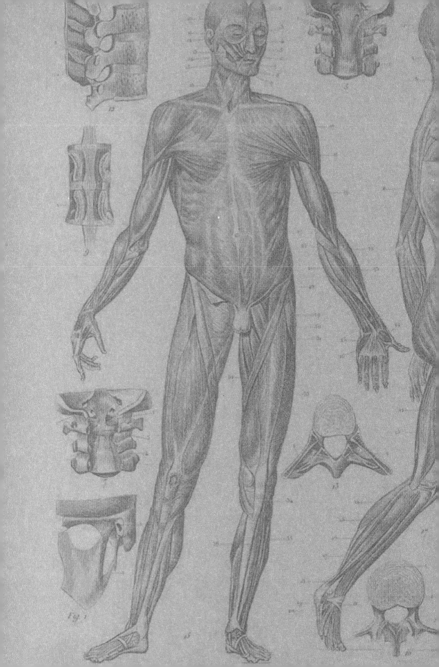

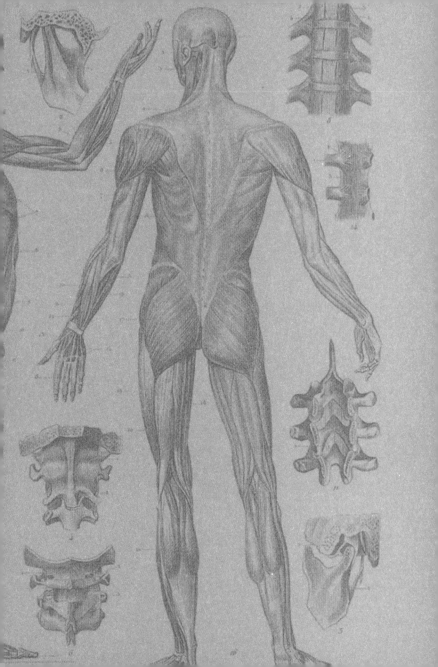

In the winter of 2000, during the first year of my medical residency, I lived in a one-room apartment facing a park, a few steps from the train station at Harvard Square.

Lived is a euphemism. I was on call every third night at the hospital—awake the whole night, admitting patients to the medical wards, writing notes, performing procedures, or caring for the acutely ill in intensive care units. The next day—*postcall*—was usually spent in a dull haze on my futon, catching up on lost sleep. The third day we named *flex*, for "flexible." Rounds were usually done by six in the evening—and the four or five hours of heady wakefulness that remained were among the most precious and private of all my possessions. I ran a three-mile circuit around the frozen Charles River as if my life depended on it, made coffee on a sputtering Keurig, and stared vacantly at the snowdrifts through my window, ruminating on the cases that I had seen that week. By the end of the first six months, I had witnessed more than a dozen deaths, including that of a young man, no older than I, who died of organ failure while awaiting a heart transplant.

. . . .

I spoke to no one, or, at least, I have no memory of speaking to anyone (I ran through a park by night, and through friends by day). "Illness reminds you that spontaneity, too, is a human right," a patient once told me. Part of the horror of hospitals is that everything happens on time: medicines arrive on schedule; the sheets are changed on schedule; the doctors round at set times; even urine is collected in a graduated pouch on a timer. Those who tend the ill also experience some of this erasure of spontaneity. Looking back, I realize that I lived for a year, perhaps two, like a clockwork human, moving from one subroutine to the next. Days folded into identical days, all set to the same rhythm. By the end of my first month, even "flex" had turned into reflex.

The only way to break the deadly monotony was to read. In the medieval story, a prisoner is sent to jail with just one book, but discovers a cosmos of a thousand books in that single volume. In my recollection, I also read only one book that year— a slim paperback collection of essays titled *The Youngest Science*—but I read it as if it were a thousand books. It became one of the most profound influences on my life in medicine.

....

The Youngest Science was subtitled *Notes of a Medicine-Watcher* and was about a medical residency in another age. Written by the physician, scientist, author, and occasional poet Lewis Thomas, it describes his tenure as a medical resident and intern in the 1930s. In 1937, having graduated from Harvard Medical School, Thomas began his internship at Boston City Hospital. It was a grueling initiation. "Rewarding might be the wrong word for it, for the salary was no money at all," Thomas wrote. "A bedroom, board, and the laundering of one's white uniform were provided by the hospital; the hours of work were all day, every day. . . . There was little need for pocket money because there was no time to spend pocket money. In any case, the interns had one sure source of spare cash: they were the principal donors of blood transfusions, at $25 a pint; two or three donations a month kept us in affluence."

Lewis Thomas entered medicine at one of the most pivotal transitional moments in its history. We tend to forget that much of "modern medicine" is, in fact, surprisingly modern: before the 1930s, you would be hard-pressed to identify a single medical intervention that had any more than a negligible impact on the course of any illness (surgery, in contrast, could have a transformative effect; think of an appendectomy for appendicitis, or an amputation for gangrene). Nearly every medical intervention could be categorized as one of three P's—placebo, palliation, and plumbing. Placebos were, of course, the most common of drugs—"medicines" that caused their effects by virtue of psychological or psychosomatic reactions in patients (elixirs for weakness and aging, or tonics for depression).

Palliative drugs, in contrast, were often genuinely effective; they included morphine, opium, alcohol, and various tinctures, poultices, and balms used to ameliorate symptoms such as itching and pain. The final category—I've loosely labeled it "plumbing"—included laxatives, purgatives, emetics, and enemas used to purge the stomach and intestines of their contents to relieve constipation and, occasionally, to disgorge poisons. These worked, although they were of limited use in most medical cases. (In an epic perversion, the tool and the therapy were often inverted. Purging was a common medical intervention in the nineteenth century not because it was particularly effective, but because it was one of the few things that doctors could actually achieve through medicines; if you had a hammer, as the saying goes, then everything looks like a nail.)

The paucity and ineffectiveness of therapeutic interventions had created what Thomas recognized as the reigning philosophy of medicine: "therapeutic nihilism." Despite the negative connotations in its name, therapeutic nihilism was arguably one of the most positive developments of early twentieth-century medicine. Recognizing the absolute uselessness—and the frank perniciousness—of most nineteenth-century medical interventions, a new generation of doctors had decided to refrain from doing much at all. Instead, luminaries such as William Osler, at Johns Hopkins, had chosen to concentrate on defining, observing, categorizing, and naming diseases, hoping that this would allow future generations to identify bona fide therapeutic interventions. Osler, for instance, hospitalized patients in medical wards in Baltimore with no other purpose, it seemed, than to watch the "natural history" of an illness unfold in real time. The all-too-human temptation to do something was purposefully stifled. (A doctor's job, Thomas once told an interviewer, "was to make a diagnosis, make a prognosis, give support and care—and not to meddle.") Osler's students didn't meddle with useless medicines; instead, they measured volumes, breaths, weights, and heights; they listened to hearts and lungs, looked at pupils dilating and contracting, abdomens growing and shrinking, neural reflexes appearing and disappearing. It seemed as if the Hippocratic oath—*First, do no harm*—had been transmuted to *First, do nothing.*

And yet, doing nothing would have a deeply cleansing effect. By the 1930s, the careful bloodletting of the past had radically altered the discipline; by observing the evolution of diseases, and by constructing models of how diseases occurred and progressed, doctors had begun to lay the foundations of a new kind of medicine.

They had recognized the cardinal features of heart failure—the gradual overloading of the body with fluid and its extrusion into the lungs, the altered sounds of the stretched, overworked heart, or the lethal disruptions of rhythm that followed. Diabetes, they had learned, was a dysfunction of the metabolism of sugar—the body's inability to move sugar from blood into tissues; that in patients with diabetic acidosis, blood became gradually saturated with glucose, yet the tissues were starved of nutrition, like the Mariner who finds water everywhere, but cannot get a drop to drink. Or that streptococcal pneumonias often followed influenza infection; that patients recovering from the flu might suddenly develop relapsing fevers and a hacking, blood-tinged cough; that through the earpiece of a stethoscope, a single lobe of the lung might be found to exhibit the characteristic dull rustling of consolidation—"like a man walking on autumn leaves," as one professor of mine described it. Or that a patient with such a pneumonia might experience two very different trajectories: either the microbe would overwhelm his physiological defenses, resulting in sepsis, organ failure, and a swift death; or, about ten days into the infection, the body would mount an exquisite immunological defense against the organism, resulting in the sudden abatement of fever and the elimination of the bacterium from the blood. Pathophysiology—the physiology of pathology—was thus constructed, observation upon observation, and it would be the platform on which modern medicine could be built.

For Thomas, the astonishing feature of medicine in the 1940s was its ability to use this information to mount genuine therapeutic interventions against diseases based on rational precepts. Once heart failure had been reconceived in terms of pump dysfunction and volume overload (a failing pump cannot move the same volume of blood through the body, and the extra volume froths back into the lungs), then an effective, albeit crude, therapy for heart failure became self-evident: removing a few pints of blood from the veins to ease the straining heart. Similarly, once the miraculous recovery from streptococcal infection had been understood as the deployment of a host immunological response, then this, too, suggested a novel therapeutic approach: transferring serum from a convalescent human or animal to a newly infected patient to supply the crucial defensive factors (later found to be antistreptococcal antibodies) to boost the host's immunological response. Here is Thomas describing the treatment for streptococcal pneumonia based on this principle: "The serum was injected, very slowly, by vein. When it worked, it worked within an hour or two. Down came the temperature, and the patient, who might have been moribund a few hours earlier, would be sleeping in good health."

Thomas wrote, "For an intern it was an opening of a new world. We had been raised to be ready for one kind of profession, and we sensed that the profession itself had changed at the moment of our entry. . . . We became convinced, overnight, that nothing lay beyond the reach of the future. Medicine was off and running." It was the birth of what Thomas called the "youngest science."

. . . .

By the time I read *The Youngest Science*, the scientific transformation of medicine had deepened even further. Take heart failure again. In 1937, Thomas wrote, the only reliable means to affect a failing heart, aside from propping up its function with extra oxygen, was to alter blood volume by inserting a needle into a vein and drawing out a hundred milliliters of fluid from the body. To a cardiologist working in the late 1990s, this would be akin to lancing an abscess using a skin cup: it might work, but it was a decidedly medieval approach. This cardiologist would now have at his disposal not one, or two, but no less than a dozen medicines to subtly modulate the volume, pressure, and rhythm of the failing heart, including diuretics, blood-pressure mediators, drugs that open channels for salt and water in kidneys, or medicines that maintain fine control on heart rhythms. Added to this were implantable defibrillators (colloquially called heart zappers) that delivered jolts of electricity to "reset" the heart should it enter a lethal rhythmic cycle. For the most intractable cases of heart failure—such as the young man whose heart muscles were destroyed, bit by bit, by the mysterious deposition of iron, like the Tin Man of Oz—even more innovative procedures exist, such as the transplantation of a whole foreign heart into the body, followed by a salvo of immunosuppressive medicines to ensure that the transplanted graft remains functional and intact in the body afterward.

....

But the more I read *The Youngest Science* that year, the more I returned to a fundamental question: Is medicine a science? If, by *science*, we are referring to the spectacular technological innovations of the past decades, then without doubt medicine qualifies. But technological innovations do not define a science; they merely prove that medicine is scient*ific*—i.e., therapeutic interventions are based on the rational precepts of pathophysiology.

Sciences have laws—statements of truth based on repeated experimental observations that describe some universal or generalizable attributes of nature. Physics is replete with such laws. Some are powerful and general, such as the law of gravitation, which describes the force of attraction between two bodies with mass anywhere in the universe. Others apply to specific conditions, such as Ohm's law, which only holds true for certain kinds of electrical circuits. In every case, however, a law distills a relationship between observable phenomena that remains true across multiple circumstances and multiple conditions. Laws are rules that nature must live by.

There are fewer laws in chemistry. Biology is the most lawless of the three basic sciences: there are few rules to begin with, and even fewer rules that are universal. Living creatures must, of course, obey the fundamental rules of physics and chemistry, but life often exists on the margins and in the interstices of these laws, bending them to their near-breaking limit. Even the elephant cannot violate the laws of thermodynamics—although its trunk, surely, must rank as one of the most peculiar means to move matter using energy.

But does the "youngest science" have laws? It seems like an odd preoccupation now, but I spent much of my medical residency seeking the laws of medicine. The criteria were simple: a "law" had to distill some universal guiding principle of medicine into a statement of truth. The law could not be borrowed from biology or chemistry; it had to be specific to the practice of medicine. In 1978, in a mordantly acerbic book called *The House of God*, the writer Samuel Shem had proposed "thirteen laws of medicine" (an example: "Law 12: if the radiology resident and the intern both see a lesion on an X-ray, then the lesion cannot be there"). But the laws that I was seeking were not attempts to skewer medical culture or highlight its perversities à la Shem; I was genuinely interested in rules, or principles, that applied to the practice of medicine at large.

Of course, these would not be laws like those of physics or chemistry. If medicine is a science at all, it is a much softer science. There is gravity in medicine, although it cannot be captured by Newton's equations. There is a half-life of grief, even if there is no instrument designed to measure it. The laws of medicine would not be described through equations, constants, or numbers. My search for the laws was not an attempt to codify or reduce the discipline into grand universals. Rather, I imagined them as guiding rules that a young doctor might teach himself as he navigates a profession that seems, at first glance, overwhelmingly unnavigable. The project began lightly—but it eventually produced some of the most serious thinking that I have ever done around the basic tenets of my discipline.

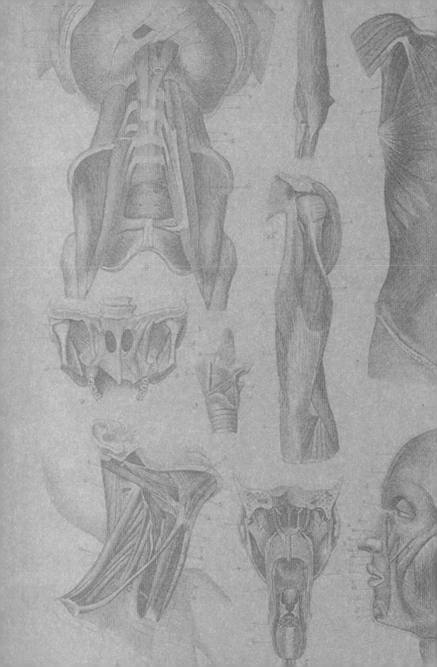

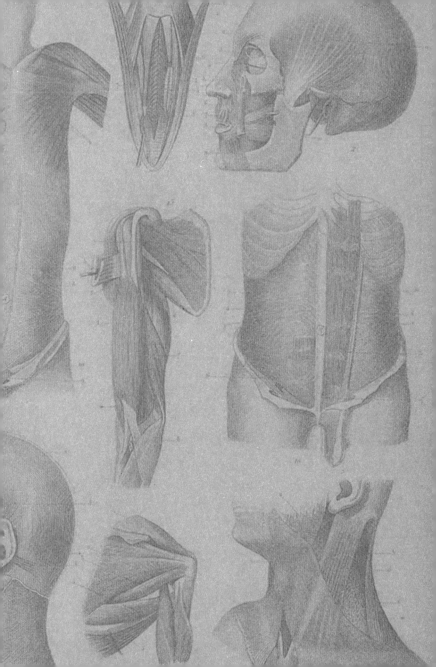

A strong intuition is much more powerful than a weak test.

I discovered the first law of medicine by chance—which is exactly as it should be since it largely concerns chance. In the spring of 2001, toward the end of my internship year, I was asked to see a man with unexplained weight loss and fatigue. He was fifty-six years old, and a resident of Beacon Hill, the tony neighborhood with brick town houses and tree-lined, cobblestone streets that abuts Massachusetts General Hospital.

Mr. Carlton—as I'll call him—was the Hill distilled to its essence. With his starched blue shirt, a jacket with elbow patches, and a silk necktie fraying just so, he suggested money, but old money, the kind that can be stuffed under blankets. There was something in his manner—a quicksilver volatility, an irritability—that I could not quite pin down. When he stood up, I noticed that the leather belt around his waist had been cinched tightly. More ominously, the muscles on the side of his forehead had begun to shrivel—a phenomenon called temporal wasting—which clearly suggested the weight loss had been recent and quite severe. He stood up to be weighed and told me that he had lost nearly twenty-six pounds over the last four months. Even the journey from the chair to the scale was like crossing an ocean. He had to sit down again afterward to catch his breath.

The most obvious culprit was cancer—some occult, hidden malignancy that was driving this severe cachexia. He had no obvious risk factors: he was not a smoker and had no suggestive family history. I ran some preliminary labs on him, but they were largely normal, save for a mild drop in his white-cell count that could be attributed to virtually anything.

Over the next four weeks, we scoured his body for signs of cancer. CAT scans were negative. A colonoscopy, looking for an occult colon cancer, revealed nothing except for an occasional polyp. He saw a rheumatologist—for the fleeting arthritic pains in his fingers—but again, nothing was diagnosed. I sent out another volley of lab tests. The technician in the blood lab complained that Mr. Carlton's veins were so pinched that she could hardly draw any blood.

For a while nothing happened. It felt like a diagnostic stalemate. More tests came back negative. Mr. Carlton was frustrated; his weight kept dropping, threatening to go all the way down to zero. Then, one evening, returning home from the hospital, I witnessed an event that changed my entire perspective on the case.

Boston is a small town—and the geography of illness tracks the geography of its neighborhoods (I'll risk admonishment here, but this is how medical interns think). To the northeast lie the Italian neighborhoods of the North End and the rough-and-tumble shipyards of Charlestown and Dorchester, with high densities of smokers and asbestos-exposed ship workers (think lung cancer, emphysema, asbestosis). To the south are desperately poor neighborhoods overrun by heroin and cocaine. Beacon Hill and Brookline, sitting somewhere in the middle, are firmly middle-class bastions, with the spectra of chronic illnesses that generally affect the middle class.

What happened that evening amounted to this: around six o'clock as I left the hospital after rounds, I saw Mr. Carlton in the lobby, by the Coffee Exchange, conversing with a man whom I had admitted months ago with a severe skin infection related to a heroin needle inserted incorrectly into a vein. The conversation could not have lasted for more than a few minutes. It may have involved something as innocuous as change for a twenty-dollar bill, or directions to the nearest ATM. But on my way home on the train, the image kept haunting me: *the Beacon Hill scion chatting with the Mission Hill addict.* There was a dissonant familiarity in their body language that I could not shake off—a violation of geography, of accent, of ancestry, of dress code, of class. By the time I reached my station, I knew the answer. Boston is a small town. It should have been obvious all along: Mr. Carlton was a heroin user. Perhaps the man at the Coffee Exchange was his sometime dealer, or an acquaintance of an acquaintance. In retrospect, I should also have listened to the blood-lab worker who had had such a hard time drawing Mr. Carlton's blood: his veins were likely scarred from habitual use.

The next week, I matter-of-factly offered Mr. Carlton an HIV test. I told him nothing of the meeting that I had witnessed. Nor did I ever confirm that he knew the man from Mission Hill. The test was strikingly positive. By the time the requisite viral-load and the CD4 counts had been completed, we had clinched the diagnosis: Mr. Carlton had AIDS.

....

I'm describing this case in such detail because it contains a crucial insight. Every diagnostic challenge in medicine can be imagined as a probability game. This is how you play the game: you assign a probability that a patient's symptoms can be explained by some pathological dysfunction—heart failure, say, or rheumatoid arthritis—and then you summon evidence to increase or decrease the probability. Every scrap of evidence—a patient's medical history, a doctor's instincts, findings from a physical examination, past experiences, rumors, hunches, behaviors, gossip—raises or lowers the probability. Once the probability tips over a certain point, you order a confirmatory test—and then you read the test in the context of the prior probability. My encounter with Mr. Carlton in the lobby of the hospital can be now reconceived as such a probability game. From my perceptual biases, I had assigned Mr. Carlton an infinitesimally low chance of HIV infection. By the end of that fateful evening, though, my corner-of-the-eye encounter had shifted that probability dramatically. The shift was enough to tip the scales, trigger the test, and reveal the ultimate diagnosis.

But this, you might object, is a strange way to diagnose an illness. What sense does it make to assess the probability of a positive test *before* a test? Why not go to the test directly? A more thoughtful internist, you might argue, would have screened a patient for HIV right away and converged swiftly on the diagnosis without fumbling along, as I had, for months.

It is here that an insight enters our discussion—and it might sound peculiar at first: *a test can only be interpreted sanely in the context of prior probabilities.* It seems like a rule taken from a Groucho Marx handbook: you need to have a glimpse of an answer before you have the glimpse of the answer (nor, for that matter, should you seek to become a member of a club that will accept you as a member).

To understand the logic behind this paradox, we need to understand that every test in medicine—any test in any field, for that matter—has a false-positive and false-negative rate. In a false positive, a test is positive even when the patient does not have the disease or abnormality (the HIV test reads positive, but you don't have the virus). In a false negative, a patient tests negative, but actually has the abnormality being screened for (you are infected, but the test is negative).

The point is this: if patients are screened without any *prior* knowledge about their risks, then the false-positive or false-negative rates can confound any attempt at diagnosis. Consider the following scenario. Suppose the HIV test has a false-positive rate of 1 in 1,000—i.e., one of out every thousand patients tests positive, even though the patient carries no infection (the actual false-positive rate has decreased since my time as an intern, but remains in this range). And suppose, further, we deploy this test in a population of patients where the prevalence of HIV infection is also 1 in 1,000. To a close approximation, for every infected patient who tests positive, there will also be one uninfected person who will also test positive. For every test that comes back positive, in short, there is only a 50 percent chance that the patient is actually positive. Such a test, we'd all agree, is not particularly useful: it only works half the time. The "more thoughtful internist" in our original scenario gains very little by ordering an HIV test on a man with no risk factors: if the *test* comes back positive, it is more likely that the test is false, rather than the infection is real. If the false-positive rate rises to 1 percent and the prevalence falls to 0.05 percent—both realistic numbers—then the chance of a positive test's being real falls to an abysmal 5 percent. The test is now wrong *95 percent* of the time.

In contrast, watch what happens if the same population is *preselected*, based on risk behaviors or exposures. Suppose our preselection strategy is so accurate that we can stratify patients as "high risk" *before* the test. Now, the up-front prevalence of infection climbs to 19 in 100, and the situation changes dramatically. For every twenty positive tests, only one is a false positive, and nineteen are true positives—an accuracy rate of 95 percent. It seems like a trick pulled out of a magician's hat: by merely changing the structure of the tested population, the same test is transformed from perfectly useless to perfectly useful. You need a strong piece of "prior knowledge"—I've loosely called it an intuition—to overcome the weakness of a test.

The "prior knowledge" that I am describing is the kind of thing that old-school doctors do very well, and that new technologies in medicine often neglect. "Prior knowledge" is what is at stake when your doctor—rather than ordering yet another echocardiogram or a stress test—asks you about whether your feet have been swelling or takes your pulse for no apparent reason. I once saw a masterful oncologist examining a patient with lung cancer. The exam proceeded quite predictably. He listened to her heart and lungs. He checked her skin for rashes. He made her walk across the room. And then, as the exam came to a close, he began to ask her a volley of bizarre questions. He fussed about his office, writing his notes, then blurted out a wrong date. She corrected him, laughing. When was the last time she had gone out with her friends? he asked. Had her handwriting changed? Was she wearing an extra pair of socks with her open-toed shoes?

Once he had finished and she had left the office, I asked him about the questions. The answer was surprisingly simple: he was screening her for depression, anxiety, sleeplessness, sexual dysfunction, neuropathy, and a host of other sequelae of her illness or its treatment. He had refined the process over so many iterations that his questions, seemingly oblique, had been sharpened into needlelike probes. A woman doesn't know what to say if you ask her if she has "neuropathy," he told me, but no one can forget putting on an extra pair of socks. It's easier to summon a date that you are specifically asked for. Picking out a blurted-out date that's wrong requires a more subtle combination of attention, memory, and cognition. None of his questions was anywhere near diagnostic or definitive; if there were positive or negative signs, he would certainly need to order confirmatory tests. But he was doing the thing that the most incisive doctors do: he was weighing evidence and making inferences. He was playing with probability.

This line of reasoning, it's worthwhile noting, is not a unique feature of any particular test. It applies not only to medicine but to any other discipline that is predicated on predictions: economics or banking, gambling or astrology. The core logic holds true whether you are trying to forecast tomorrow's weather or seeking to predict rises and falls in the stock market. It is a universal feature of *all* tests.

....

The man responsible for this strange and illuminating idea was neither a doctor nor a scientist by trade. Born in Hertfordshire in 1702, Thomas Bayes was a clergyman and philosopher who served as the minister at the chapel in Tunbridge Wells, near London. He published only two significant papers in his lifetime—the first, a defense of God, and the second, a defense of Newton's theory of calculus (it was a sign of the times that in 1732, a clergyman found no cognitive dissonance between these two efforts). His best-known work—on probability theory—was not published during his lifetime and was only rediscovered decades after his death.

The statistical problem that concerned Bayes requires a sophisticated piece of mathematical reasoning. Most of Bayes's mathematical compatriots were concerned with problems of pure statistics: If you have a box of twenty-five white balls and seventy-five black balls, say, what is the chance of drawing two black balls in a row? Bayes, instead, was concerned with a converse conundrum—the problem of knowledge acquisition from observed realities. If you draw two black balls in a row from a box containing a mix of balls, he asked, what can you say about the composition of white versus black balls in the box? What if you draw two white and one black ball in a row? How does your assessment of the contents of the box change?

Perhaps the most striking illustration of Bayes's theorem comes from a riddle that a mathematics teacher that I knew would pose to his students on the first day of their class. Suppose, he would ask, you go to a roadside fair and meet a man tossing coins. The first toss lands "heads." So does the second.

And the third, fourth . . . and so forth, for twelve straight tosses. What are the chances that the next toss will land "heads"? Most of the students in the class, trained in standard statistics and probability, would nod knowingly and say: 50 percent. But even a child knows the real answer: *it's the coin that is rigged*. Pure statistical reasoning cannot tell you the answer to the question— but common sense does. The fact that the coin has landed "heads" twelve times tells you more about its future chances of landing "heads" than any abstract formula. If you fail to use prior information, you will inevitably make foolish judgments about the future. *This is the way we intuit the world*, Bayes argued. There is no absolute knowledge; there is only conditional knowledge. History repeats itself—and so do statistical patterns. The past is the best guide to the future.

It is easy to appreciate the theological import of this line of reasoning. Standard probability theory asks us to predict consequences from abstract knowledge: Knowing God's vision, what can you predict about Man? But Bayes's theorem takes the more pragmatic and humble approach to inference. It is based on real, observable knowledge: Knowing Man's world, Bayes asks, what can you guess about the mind of God?

. . . .

How might this apply to a medical test? The equations described by Bayes teach us how to interpret a test given our prior knowledge of risk and prevalence: *If* a man has a history of drug addiction, and *if* drug addicts have a higher prevalence of HIV infection, then what is the chance that a positive test is real? A test is not a Delphic oracle, Bayes reminds us; it is not a predictor of perfect truths. It is, rather, a machine that modifies probabilities. It takes information in and puts information out. We feed it an "input probability" and it gives us an "output probability." If we feed it garbage, then it will inevitably spit garbage out.

The peculiar thing about the "garbage in, garbage out" rule is that we are quick to apply it to information or computers, but are reluctant to apply it to medical tests. Take PSA testing, for instance. Prostate cancer is an age-related cancer: the incidence climbs dramatically as a man ages. If you test every man over the age of forty with a PSA test, the number of false positives will doubtless overwhelm the number of true positives. Thousands of needless biopsies and confirmatory tests will be performed, each adding complications, frustration, and cost. If you use the same test on men above sixty, the yield might increase somewhat, but the false-positive and -negative rates might still be forbidding. Add more data—family history, risk factors, genetics, or a change in PSA value over time—and the probability of a truly useful test keeps getting refined. There is no getting away from this logic. Yet, demands for indiscriminate PSA testing to "screen" for prostate cancer keep erupting among patients and advocacy groups.

The force of Bayes's logic has not diminished as medical information has expanded; it has only become more powerful. Should a woman with a mutant BRCA1 gene have a double mastectomy? "Yes" and "no" are both foolish answers. The presence of a BRCA1 mutation is well known to increase the risk of ovarian or breast cancer—but the actual risk varies vastly from person to person. One woman might develop a lethal, rapidly growing breast cancer at thirty; another woman might only develop an indolent variant in her eighties. A Bayesian analyst would ask you to seek more information: Did a woman's mother or grandmother have breast cancer? At what age? What do we know about her previous risks—genes, exposures, environments? Are any of the risks modifiable?

If you scan the daily newspapers to identify the major "controversies" simmering through medicine, they inevitably concern Bayesian analysis, or a fundamental lack of understanding of Bayesian theory. Should a forty-year-old woman get a mammogram? Well, unless we can modify the prior probability of her having breast cancer, chances are that we will pick up more junk than real cases of cancer. What if we invented an incredibly sophisticated blood test to detect Ebola? Should we screen all travelers at the airport using such a test and thereby prevent the spread of a lethal virus into the United States? Suppose I told you, further, that *every person who had Ebola tested positive with this test*, and the only drawback was a modest 5 percent false-positive rate. On first glance, it seems like a no-brainer. But watch what happens with Bayesian analysis. Assume that 1 percent of travelers are actually infected with Ebola—a hefty fraction. If a man tests positive at the airport, what is the actual chance that he is infected? Most people guess some number between 50 and 90 percent. The actual answer is about 16 percent. If the actual prevalence of infection among travelers drops to 0.1 percent, a more realistic fraction, then the chance of a positive test being real drops to a staggering 2 percent. In other words, 98 percent of tests will be false, and our efforts will be overwhelmed trying to hunt for the two cases that are real out of a hundred.

Can't we devise tests of such accuracy and consistency that we can escape the dismal mathematical orbit of Bayes's theorem? What if we could decrease the false-positive rate to such a low number that we would no longer need to bother with prior probabilities? The "screen everyone for everything" approach—Dr. McCoy's handheld all-body scanner in *Star Trek*—works if we have infinite resources and absolutely perfect tests, but it begins to fail when resources and time are finite. Perhaps in the future we can imagine a doctor who doesn't have to take a careful history, feel the contours of your pulse, ask questions about your ancestors, inquire about your recent trip to a new planetary system, or watch the rhythm of your gait as you walk out of the office. Perhaps all the uncertain, unquantifiable, inchoate priors—inferences, as I've called them loosely—will become obsolete. But by then, medicine will have changed. We will be orbiting some new world, and we'll have to learn new laws for medicine.

····

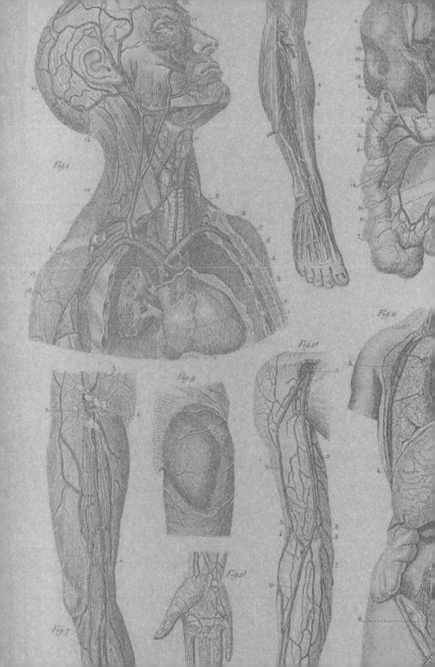

Fig.1

Fig.9

Fig.7

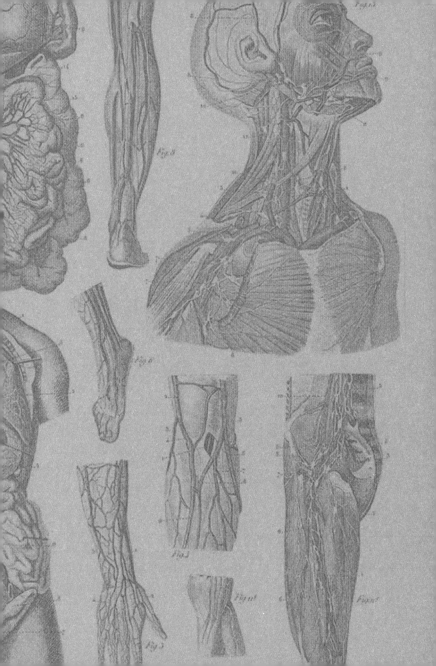

"Normals" teach us rules; "outliers" teach us laws.

Tycho Brahe was the most famous astronomer of his time. Born to a wealthy family in Scania, Denmark (now a part of Sweden), in 1546, Brahe became keenly interested in astronomy as a young man and soon began a systematic study of the motion of planets. His key discovery—that the stars were not "tailless comets" that had been pinned to an invisible canopy in the heavens, but were massive bodies radiating light from vast distances in space—shot him to instant fame. Granted an enormous, windswept island estate on the Øresund strait by the king, Brahe launched the construction of a gigantic observatory to understand the organization of the cosmos.

In Brahe's time, the most widely accepted view of the universe was one that had been proposed centuries earlier by the Greek astronomer Ptolemy: the earth sat at the center of the solar system, and the planets, sun, and moon revolved around it. Ptolemy's theory satisfied the ancient human desire to sit at the center of the solar system, but it could not explain the observed motion of the planets and the moon using simple orbits. To explain those movements, Ptolemy had to resort to bizarrely convoluted orbital paths, in which some planets circled the earth, but also moved in smaller "epicycles" around themselves, like spinning dervishes that traced chains of rings around a central ring. The model was riddled with contradictions and exceptions—but there was nothing better. In 1512, an eccentric Prussian polymath named Nicolaus Copernicus published a rough pamphlet claiming—heretically—that the *sun* sat at the center of the planets, and the earth revolved around it. But even

Copernicus's model could not explain the movements of the planets. His orbits were strictly circular—and the predicted positions of the planets deviated so far from the observed positions that it was easy to write it all off as nonsense.

Brahe recognized the powerful features of Copernicus's model—it simplified many of Ptolemy's problems—but he still could not bring himself to believe it (the earth is a "hulking, lazy body, unfit for motion," he wrote). Instead, in an attempt to make the best of both cosmological worlds, Brahe proposed a hybrid model of the universe, with the earth still at the center and the sun moving around it—but with the other planets revolving around the sun.

Brahe's model was spectacular. His strength as a cosmologist was the exquisite accuracy of his measurements, and his model worked perfectly for nearly every measured orbit. The rules were beautiful, except for a pesky planet called Mars. Mars just would not fit. It was the outlier, the aberration, the grain of sand in the eye of Tychonian cosmology. If you carefully follow Mars on the horizon, it tracks a peculiar path—pitching forward at first and then tacking *backward* in space before resuming a forward motion again. This phenomena—called the retrograde motion of Mars—did not make sense in either Ptolemy's or Brahe's model. Fed up with Mars's path across the evening sky, Brahe assigned the problem to an indigent, if exceptionally ambitious, young assistant named Johannes Kepler, a young mathematician from Germany with whom he had a stormy, on-again, off-again relationship. Brahe quite possibly threw Kepler the "Mars problem" to keep him distracted with an insoluble conundrum of little value. Perhaps Kepler, too, would be stuck cycling two steps forward and five steps back, leaving Brahe to ponder real questions of cosmological importance.

Kepler, however, did not consider Mars peripheral: if a planetary model was real, it had to explain the movements of all the planets, not just the convenient ones. He studied the motion of Mars obsessively. He managed to retain some of Brahe's astronomical charts even after Brahe's death, fending off rapacious heirs for nearly a decade while he pored carefully through the borrowed data. He tried no less than forty different models to explain the retrograde motion of Mars. The drunken "doubling back" of the planet would not fit. Then the answer came to him in an inspired flash: the orbits of all the planets were not circles, but *ellipses* around the sun. All the planets, including Mars, orbit the sun in concentric ellipses. Seen from the earth, Mars moves "backward" in the same sense that one train appears to pitch backward when another train overtakes it on a parallel track. What Brahe had dismissed as an aberration was the most important piece of information needed to understand the organization of the cosmos. The exception to the rule, it turned out, was crucial to the formulation of Keppler's Law.

....

In 1908, when psychiatrists encountered children who were withdrawn, self-absorbed, emotionally uncommunicative, and often prone to repetitive behaviors, they classified the disease as a strange variant of schizophrenia. But the diagnosis of schizophrenia would not fit. As child psychiatrists studied these children over time, it became clear that this illness was quite distinct from schizophrenia, although certain features overlapped. Children with this disease seemed to be caught in a labyrinth of their own selves, unable to escape. In 1912, the Swiss psychiatrist Paul Eugen Bleuler coined a new word to describe the illness: *autism*—from the Greek word for "self."

For a few decades, psychiatrists studied families and children with autism, trying to make sense of the disease. They noted that the disease ran in families, often coursing through multiple generations, and that children with autism tended to have older parents, especially older fathers. But no systematic model for the illness yet existed. Some scientists argued that the disease was related to abnormal neural development. But in the 1960s, from the throes of psychoanalytical and behavioral thinking, a powerful new theory took root and held fast: autism was the result of parents who were emotionally cold to their children.

Almost everything about the theory seemed to fit. Observed carefully, the parents of children with autism did seem remote and detached from their children. That children learn behaviors by mirroring the actions of their parents was well established—and it seemed perfectly plausible that they might imitate their emotional responses as well. Animals deprived of their parents in experimental situations develop maladaptive, repetitive behaviors—and so, children with such parents might also develop these symptoms. By the early 1970s, this theory had hardened into the "refrigerator mom" hypothesis. Refrigerator moms, unable to thaw their own selves, had created icy, withdrawn, socially awkward children, resulting ultimately in autism.

The refrigerator mom theory caught the imagination of psychiatry—could there be a more potent mix than sexism and a mysterious illness?—and unleashed a torrent of therapies for autism. Children with autism were treated with electrical shocks, with "attachment therapies," with hallucinogenic drugs to "warm" them to the world, with behavioral counseling to correct their maladapted parenting. One psychiatrist proposed a radical "parent-ectomy"—akin to a surgical mastectomy for breast cancer, except here the diseased parent was to be excised from the child's life.

Yet, the family history of autism would not fit the model. It was hard to imagine emotional refrigeration, whatever that was, running through multiple generations; no one had documented such an effect. Nor was it simple to explain away the striking incidence of autism in children of older male parents.

We now know that autism has little to with "refrigerator moms." When geneticists examined the risk of autism between identical twins, they found a striking rate of concordance— between 50 and 80 percent in most studies—strongly suggesting a genetic cause of the illness. In 2012, biologists began to analyze the genomes of children with so-called spontaneous autism. In these cases, the siblings and parents of the child do not have the disease, but a child develops it—allowing biologists to compare and contrast the genome of a child with that of his or her parents. These gene-sequencing studies uncovered dozens of genes that differed between parents without autism and children with autism, again strongly suggesting a genetic cause. Many of the mutations cluster around genes that have to do with the brain and neural development. Many of them result in altered neurodevelopmental anatomies—brain circuits that seem abnormally organized.

In retrospect, we now know that the behavior of the mothers of autistic children was not the cause of autism; it was the effect—an emotional response to a child who produces virtually no emotional response. There are, in short, no refrigerator moms. There are only neurodevelopmental pathways that, lacking appropriate signals and molecules, have gone cold.

....

The moral and medical lessons from this story are even more relevant today. Medicine is in the midst of a vast reorganization of fundamental principles. Most of our models of illness are hybrid models; past knowledge is mishmashed with present knowledge. These hybrid models produce the illusion of a systematic understanding of a disease—but the understanding is, in fact, incomplete. Everything seems to work spectacularly, until one planet begins to move backward on the horizon. We have invented many rules to understand normalcy—but we still lack a deeper, more unified understanding of physiology and pathology.

This is true for even for the most common and extensively studied diseases—cancer, heart disease, and diabetes. If cancer is a disease in which genes that control cell division are mutated, thus causing unbridled cellular growth, then why do the most exquisitely targeted inhibitors of cell division fail to cure most cancers? If type 2 diabetes results from the insensitivity of tissues to insulin signaling, then why does adding extra insulin reverse many, but not all, features of the disease? Why do certain autoimmune diseases cluster together in some people, while others have only one variant? Why do patients with some neurological diseases, such as Parkinson's disease, have a reduced risk of cancer? These "outlying" questions are the Mars problems of medicine: they point to systematic flaws in our understanding, and therefore to potentially new ways of organizing the cosmos.

Every outlier represents an opportunity to refine our understanding of illness. In 2009, a young cancer scientist named David Solit in New York set off on a research project that, at first glance, might seem like a young scientist's folly. It is a long-established fact in the world of cancer pharmacology that nine out of ten drugs in clinical development are doomed to fail. In pharmaceutical lingo, this phenomenon is called the valley of death: a new drug moves smoothly along in its early phase of clinical development, seemingly achieving all its scientific milestones, yet it inevitably falters and dies during an actual clinical trial. In some cases, a trial has to be stopped because of unanticipated toxicities. In other cases, the medicine provokes no response, or the response is not durable. Occasionally, a trial shows a striking response, but it is unpredictable and fleetingly rare. Only 1 woman in a trial of 1,000 women might experience a near complete disappearance of all the metastatic lesions of breast cancer—while 999 women experience no response. One patient with widely spread melanoma might live for fifteen years, while the rest of the cohort has died by the seventh month of the trial.

The trouble with such "exceptional responders," as Solit called them, was that they had traditionally been ignored, brushed off as random variations, attributed to errors in diagnosis or ascribed, simply, to extraordinary good fortune. The catchphrase attached to these case histories carried the stamp of ultimate scientific damnation: *single patient anecdotes* (of all words, scientists find the word *anecdote* particularly poisonous since it refers to a subjective memory). Medical journals have long refused to publish these reports. At scientific conferences when such cases were described, researchers generally rolled their eyes and avoided the topic. When the trials ended, these responders were formally annotated as "outliers," and the drug was quietly binned.

But Solit wanted to understand these rare responses. These "exceptional responders," he reasoned, might have some peculiar combination of factors—genes, behaviors, risk factors, environmental exposures—that had made them respond so briskly and durably. He decided to use the latest medical tools to understand their responses as deeply and comprehensively as possible. He had inverted a paradigm: rather than spending an enormous effort trying to figure out why a drug had commonly failed, as most of his colleagues might have, he would try to understand why it had occasionally succeeded. He would try to map the landscape of the valley of death—not by querying all those who had fallen into it, but by asking the one or two patients who had clambered out.

In 2012, Solit's team published the first analysis of one such trial. Forty-four patients with advanced bladder cancer had been treated with a new drug called everolimus. The results had been uniformly disappointing. Some tumors may have shrunk a little, but none of the patients had showed a striking response. Then, in mid-April 2010, there was patient 45—a seventy-three-year-old woman with tumors filling her entire abdomen and invading her kidneys and lymph nodes. She started the medicine that month. Within weeks, her tumors had begun to involute. The mass invading the kidney necrosed and disappeared. Fifteen months later, when her CAT scans were checked again, her doctors had to squint hard to see any visible signs of tumor in her abdomen.

Solit focused on just that case. Reasoning that genes were likely involved, he pulled out patient 45's tumor sample from the freezer and sequenced every gene to find the ones that were mutated (in most human cancers, between 10 to 150 genes can be mutated). The woman's tumor had 140 mutations. Of all those, two stood out: one in a gene named TSC1 and another in a gene named NF2. Both these genes had been suspected to modulate the response to everolimus, but before Solit, no one had found formal proof of the link in human patients.

But this was still a "single patient anecdote"; scientists would still roll their eyes. Solit's team now returned to the original trial and sequenced the same genes in the larger cohort of patients. A pattern emerged immediately. Four other patients who had mutations in the TSC1 gene had shown modest responses, while none of the other patients, with mutations in other genes but not in TSC1, had shown even a sliver of a response. Via just one variable—the mutation in the TSC1 gene—you could segregate the trial into moderate or strong responders versus nonresponders. "Single patient anecdotes are often dismissed," Solit wrote. But here, exactly such an anecdote had turned out to be a portal to a new scientific direction. In a future trial, a cohort of patients might be sequenced *up front*, and only those with mutations in the TSC1 gene might be treated with the drug. Perhaps more important, the relationship between the gene and the susceptibility of the tumor cells opened a new series of scientific investigations into the mechanism for this selective vulnerability, leading to yet new trials and novel drugs.

But is it a *law* of medicine that such outliers will provide the most informative pieces of data in our attempt to revamp the core of our discipline? In Lewis Thomas's time, such a law would have made no sense: there was nothing to "outlie." The range of medical and surgical interventions was so severely limited that any assessment of variations in response was useless; if every patient with heart failure was destined to die, then it made little sense discriminating one from another (and even if some survived long term, no tools existed to investigate them). But this is precisely what has changed: pieces of data that do not fit our current models of illness have become especially important not only because we are reassessing the nature of our knowledge, but also because we are generating more such pieces of data every day. Think about the vast range of medicines and surgical procedures not as therapeutic interventions but as investigational probes. Think of every drug as a chemical tool—a molecular scalpel—that perturbs human physiology. Aspirin flicks off a switch in the inflammatory system. Lipitor tightens a screw on cholesterol metabolism. The more such investigational probes we use, the more likely we are to alter physiology. And the more we alter physiology, the more we will find variations in response, and thereby discover its hidden, inner logic.

. . . .

One morning in the spring of 2015, I led a group of medical students at Columbia University on what I called "outlier rounds." We were hunting for variant responses to wound healing. Most patients with surgical incisions heal their wounds in a week. But what about the few patients whose wounds don't heal? We moved from room to room across the hospital, trying to find cases where postsurgical wounds had failed to heal. Most of these were predictable—elderly patients with complex surgical incisions, or diabetics, who are known to heal poorly. But after about nine such cases, we entered the room of a young woman recovering from an abdominal procedure whose incision was still raw and unhealed. The students looked puzzled. Nothing about this woman, or her incision, seemed any different from the hundreds of others that had healed perfectly. After a long pause they began to ask questions. One of them asked about her family history: Had anyone else in her family had a similar experience? Another wondered if he might swab the tissue to check for unusual, indolent infections. The orthodox models of wound healing were coming apart at the seams, I suspected, and a novel way of thinking about an old problem was being born.

We have spent much of our time in medicine dissecting and understanding what we might call the "inlier" problem. By "inliers," I am referring to the range of normalcy; we have compiled a vast catalog of normal physiological parameters: blood pressure, height, body mass, metabolic rate. Even pathological states are described in terms that have been borrowed from normalcy: there is an average diabetic, a typical case of heart failure, and a standard responder to cancer chemotherapy.

But we have little understanding of what makes an individual lie outside the normal range. "Inliers" allow us to create rules —but "outliers" act as portals to understand deeper laws. The standard formula—height (in cms) – 100 = average weight plus 10 percent (in kgs)—is a rule that works for most of the human population. But it takes a single encounter with a person with genetic dwarfism to know that there are genes that control this relationship and that mutations can disrupt it quite acutely.

In his 1934 book, *The Logic of Scientific Discovery*, the philosopher Karl Popper proposed a crucial criterion for distinguishing a scientific system from an unscientific one. The fundamental feature of a scientific system, Popper argued, is not that its propositions are verifiable, but that its propositions are *falsifiable*—i.e., every theory carries an inherent possibility of proving it false. A theory or proposition can only be judged "scientific" if it carries within it a prediction or observation that will prove it false. Theories that fail to generate such "falsifiable" conjectures are not scientific. If medicine is to become a bona fide science, then we will have to take up every opportunity to falsify its models, so that they can be replaced by new ones.

. . . .

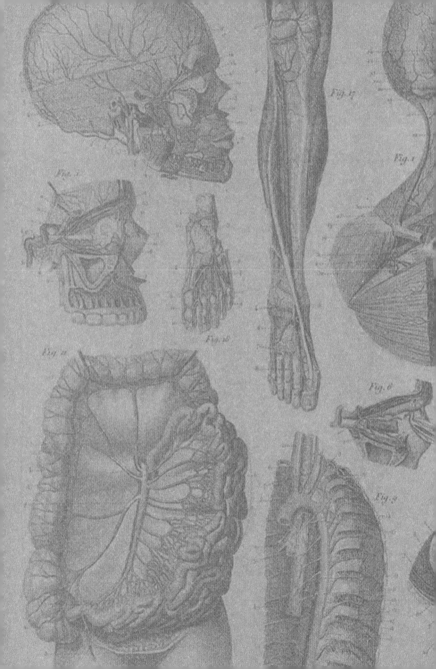

Fig. 7.

Fig. 17.

Fig. 1.

Fig. 16.

Fig. 11.

Fig. 6.

Fig. 9.

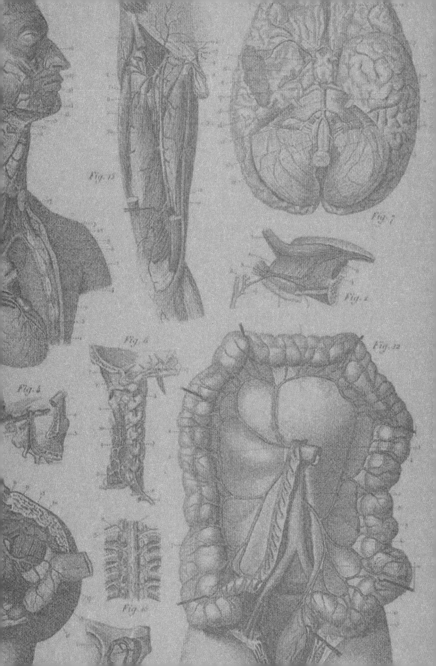

Fig. 13

Fig. 7

Fig. 2

Fig. 6

Fig. 12

Fig. 4

Fig. 10

For every perfect medical experiment, there is a perfect human bias.

In the summer of 2003, I finished my three-year residency in internal medicine and began a fellowship in oncology. It was an exhilarating time. The Human Genome Project had laid the foundation for the new science of genomics—the study of the entire genome. Although frequent criticism of the project appeared in the media—it had not lived up to its promises, some complained—it was nothing short of a windfall for cancer biology. Cancer is a genetic disease, an illness caused by mutations in genes. Until that time, most scientists had examined cancer cells one gene at a time. With the advent of new technologies to examine thousands of genes in parallel, the true complexity of cancers was becoming evident. The human genome has about twenty-four thousand genes in total. In some cancers, up to a hundred and twenty genes were altered—one in every two hundred genes—while in others, only two or three genes were mutated. (Why do some cancers carry such complexity, while others are genetically simpler? Even the questions—not just the answers—thrown up by the genome-sequencing project were unexpected.)

More important, the capacity to examine thousands of genes in parallel, without making any presuppositions about the mutant genes, allowed researchers to find novel, previously unknown genetic associations with cancer. Some of the newly discovered mutations in cancer were truly unexpected: the genes did not control growth directly, but affected the metabolism of nutrients or chemical modifications of DNA. The transformation has been likened to the difference between measuring one point in space versus looking at an entire landscape—but it was more. Looking at cancer before genome sequencing was looking at the known unknown. With genome sequencing at hand, it was like encountering the unknown unknown.

Much of the excitement around the discovery of these genes was driven by the idea that these could open new vistas for cancer treatment. If cancer cells were dependent on the mutant genes for their survival or growth—"addicted" to the mutations, as biologists liked to describe it—then targeting these addictions with specific molecules might force cancer cells to die. The battle-ax chemical poisons of cellular growth would become obsolete at last. The most spectacular example of one such drug, Gleevec, for a variant of leukemia, had galvanized the entire field. I still recall the first patient whom I treated with Gleevec, a fifty-six-year-old man whose bone marrow had been so eaten by leukemia that he had virtually no platelets left and would bleed profusely from every biopsy that we performed. A fellow had to meet Mr. K with a brick-size pack of sterile gauze pads in the exam room and press on his biopsy site for half an hour to prevent bleeding. About four weeks after he started treatment with Gleevec, it was my turn to perform his biopsy. I came prepared with the requisite armfuls of gauze, dreading the half-hour ordeal—except when I withdrew the needle, the wound stopped bleeding by itself. Through that nick of the skin, its edges furling with a normal-looking clot, I could see the birth of a revolution in cancer treatment.

Around the first week of my fellowship, I learned that another such drug, a molecular cousin of Gleevec's, was being tested in our hospital for a different form of cancer. The drug had shown promising effects in animal models and in early human experiments—and an early trial was forging ahead with human patients.

I had inherited a group of patients on the trial from a former fellow who had graduated from the program. Even a cursory examination of the trial patients on my roster indicated a spectacular response rate. One woman, with a massive tumor in her belly, found the masses melting away in a few weeks. Another patient had a dramatic reduction in pain from his metastasis. The other fellows, too, were witnessing similarly dramatic responses in their patients. We spoke reverentially about the drug, its striking response rate, and how it might change the landscape for the treatment of cancer.

Yet six months later, the overall results of the study revealed a surprising disappointment. Far from the 70 or 80 percent response rates that we had been expecting from our data, the overall rate was an abysmal 15 percent. The mysterious discrepancy made no sense, but the reason behind it became evident over the next few weeks when we looked deeply at the data. The oncology fellowship runs for three years, and every graduating batch of fellows passes on some patients from his or her roster to the new batch and assigns the rest to the more experienced attending physicians in the hospital. Whether a patient gets passed on to a fellow or an attending doctor is a personal decision. The only injunction is that a patient who get reassigned to a new fellow must be a case of "educational value."

In fact, every patient moved to the new fellows was a drug

responder, while all patients shunted to the attending physicians were nonresponders. Concerned that the new fellows would be unable to handle the more complex medical needs of men and women with no drug response—patients with the most treatment-resistant, recalcitrant variants of the disease—the graduating fellows had moved all the nonresponding patients to more experienced attending physicians. The assignment had no premeditated bias, yet the simple desire to help patients had sharply distorted the experiment.

....

Every science suffers from human biases. Even as we train massive machines to collect, store, and manipulate data for us, humans are the final observers, interpreters, and arbiters of that data. In medicine, the biases are particularly acute for two reasons. The first is hope: we *want* our medicines to work. Hope is a beautiful thing in medicine—its most tender center—but it is also the most dangerous. Few stories involving the mix of hope and illusion in medicine are more tragic, or more long-drawn, than that of the radical mastectomy.

By the early 1900s, during the brisk efflorescence of modern surgery, surgeons had devised meticulous operations to remove malignant tumors from the breast. Many women with cancer were cured by these surgical "extirpations"—yet, despite surgery, some women still relapsed with metastasis all over their bodies. This postsurgical relapse preoccupied great surgical minds. In Baltimore, the furiously productive surgeon William Halsted argued that malignant tissue left behind during the original surgery caused this relapse. He described breast-cancer surgery as an "unclean operation." Scattered scraps of tumor left behind by the surgeon, he argued, were the reason for the metastatic spread.

Halsted's hypothesis was logically coherent—but incorrect. For most women with breast cancer, the real reason for postsurgical relapse was not the local outgrowth of remnant scraps of malignant tissue. Rather, the cancer had migrated out of the breast long *before* surgery. Cancer cells, contrary to Halsted's expectations, did not circle in orderly metastatic parabolas around the original tumor; their spread through the body was more capricious and unpredictable. But Halsted was haunted by the "unclean operation." To test his theory of the local spread of cancer, he amputated not just the breast, but a vast mass of underlying tissue, including the muscles that move the arm and the shoulders and the deep lymph nodes in the chest, all in an effort to "cleanse" the site of the operation.

Halsted called the procedure a *radical* mastectomy, using the word *radical* in its original meaning from the Latin word for "root"; his aggressive mastectomy was meant to pull cancer out by its roots from the body. In time, though, the word itself would metastasize in meaning and transform into one of the most inscrutable sources of bias. Halsted's students—and women with breast cancer—came to think of the word *radical* in its second meaning: "brazen, innovative, bold." What surgeon or woman, faced with a lethal, relapsing disease, would choose the *non*radical mastectomy? Untested and uncontested, a theory became a law: no surgeon was willing to run a trial for a surgical operation that he *knew* would work. Halsted's proposition ossified into surgical doctrine. Cutting more had to translate into curing more.

Yet women relapsed—not occasionally, either, but in large numbers. In the 1940s, a small band of insurgent surgeons—most prominently Geoffrey Keynes in London—tried to challenge the core logic of the radical mastectomy, but to little avail. In 1980, nearly eight decades after Halsted's first operation, a randomized trial comparing radical mastectomy with a more conservative surgery was formally launched. (Bernie Fisher, the surgeon leading the trial, wrote, "In God we trust. All others must bring data.") Even that trial barely limped to its conclusion. Captivated by the logic and bravura of radical surgery, American surgeons were so reluctant to put the procedure to test that enrollment in the control arm faltered. Surgeons from Canada and other nations had to be persuaded to help complete the study.

The results were strikingly negative. Women with the radical procedure suffered a host of debilitating complications, but received no benefits: their chance of relapsing with metastatic disease was identical to that of women treated with more conservative surgery, coupled with local radiation. Breast cancer patients had been ground in the crucible of radical surgery for no real reason. The result was so destabilizing to the field that the trial was revisited in the 1990s, and again in 2000; more than two decades later, there was still no difference in outcome. It is hard to measure the full breadth of its effects, but roughly one hundred thousand to five hundred thousand women were treated with radical mastectomies between 1900 and 1985. The procedure is rarely, if ever, performed today.

....

In retrospect, the sources of bias in radical surgery are easy to spot: a powerful surgeon obsessed with innovation, a word that mutated in meaning, a generation of women forced to trust a physician's commands, and a culture of perfection that was often resistant to criticism. But other sources of bias in medicine are far more difficult to identify because they are more subtle. Unlike in virtually any of the other sciences, in medicine the subject—i.e., the patient—is not passive, but an active participant in an experiment. In the atomic world, Heisenberg's uncertainty principle holds that the position and momentum of a particle cannot simultaneously be measured with absolute accuracy. If you send a wave of light to measure the position of a particle, Heisenberg reasoned, then the wave's hitting the particle changes its momentum, and thereby its position, and so forth ad infinitum; you cannot measure both with absolute certainty. Medicine has its own version of "Heisenbergian" uncertainty: when you enroll a patient in a study, you inevitably alter the nature of the patient's psyche and, therefore, alter the study. The device used to measure the subject transforms the nature of the subject.

The active psyche of a patient, for instance, makes it particularly treacherous to run studies or trials that depend on memory. In 1993, a Harvard researcher named Edward Giovannucci set out to determine whether high-fat diets altered the risk of breast cancer. He identified a set of women with breast cancer and an age-matched cohort without breast cancer, then asked each group about their dietary habits over the last decade. The survey produced a pronounced signal: women with breast cancer were much more likely to have consumed diets higher in fat.

But this study had a twist: the women in Giovannucci's study had also completed a survey of their diets nearly a decade *before* this study, and the data had safely been stored away in a computer. When the two surveys were compared, in women without breast cancer, the actual diet and the recalled diet were largely identical. In women with breast cancer, however, the actual diet had no excess of fat. Only the "remembered" diet was high in fat. These women had unconsciously searched their memories for a cause of their cancers and had invented a culprit: their own bad habits. What better blame than self-blame?

But don't prospective, controlled, randomized, double-blind studies eliminate all these biases? The very existence of such a study—in which both control and experimental groups are randomly assigned, patients are treated prospectively and both doctors and patients are ignorant of the treatment—is a testament to how seriously medicine takes its own biases, and what contortions we must perform to guard against them (in few other scientific disciplines are such drastic measures used to eliminate systematic biases). The importance of such studies cannot be overemphasized. Several medical treatments thought to be deeply beneficial to patients based on strong anecdotal evidence, or decades of nonrandomized studies, were ultimately proved to be *harmful* based on randomized studies. These include, among other examples, the use of high-dose oxygen therapy for neonates, antiarrhythmic drugs after heart attacks, and hormone-replacement therapy in women.

Yet even that desperate experimental contortion cannot eliminate the subtlest of biases. It's the Heisenbergian principle at work again: when patients are enrolled in a study, they are inevitably affected by that enrollment. A man's decision to *enroll* in a study to measure the effect of exercise on diabetic management, say, is an active decision. It means that he participates in the medical process, follows certain instructions, or lives in particular neighborhoods with accessible health care and so forth. It might mean that he belongs to a certain race or ethnic group or a particular socioeconomic class. A randomized study might make particular conclusions about the effectiveness of a medicine—but in truth it has only judged that effectiveness in the subset of people who were randomized. The power of the experiment is critically dependent on its strong limits—and this is the very thing that makes it limited. The experiment may be perfect, but whether it is *generalizable* is a question.

The reverential status of randomized, controlled trials in medicine is its own source of bias. The BCG vaccine against tuberculosis was shown to have a potent protective effect in a randomized trial, but the effectiveness of the vaccine seems to decrease almost linearly as we move in latitude from the North to the South—where, incidentally, TB is the most prevalent (we still don't understand the basis for this effect, although genetic variation is the most obvious culprit). These distortions—call them heuristic biases—are not peripheral to the practice of medicine. Virtually every day I'm asked to decide whether a particular drug will work for a patient—an African-American man, say—when the trial was run on a population of predominantly white men in Kansas. Women are notoriously underrepresented in randomized studies. In fact, female *mice* are notoriously underrepresented in laboratory studies. Extracting medical wisdom from a randomized study thus involves much more than blithely reading the last line of the study published in some august medical journal. It involves human perception, arbitration, and interpretation—and hence involves bias.

The advent of new medical technologies will not diminish bias. They will amplify it. More human arbitration and interpretation will be needed to make sense of studies—and thus more biases will be introduced. Big data is not the solution to the bias problem; it is merely a source of more subtle (or even bigger) biases.

Perhaps the simplest way to tackle the bias problem is to confront it head-on and incorporate it into the very definition of medicine. The romantic view of medicine, particularly popular in the nineteenth century, is of the doctor as a "disease hunter" (in 1926, Paul de Kruif's book *Microbe Hunters* ignited the imagination of an entire generation). But most doctors don't really hunt diseases these days. The greatest clinicians who I know seem to have a sixth sense for biases. They understand, almost instinctively, when prior bits of scattered knowledge apply to their patients—but, more important, when they don't apply to their patients. They understand the importance of data and trials and randomized studies, but are thoughtful enough to resist their seductions. What doctors really hunt is bias.

....

Priors. Outliers. Biases. That all three laws of medicine involve limits and constraints on human knowledge is instructive. Lewis Thomas would not have predicted this stickiness of uncertainties and constraints; the future of medicine that Thomas had imagined was quite different. "The mechanization of scientific medicine is here to stay," he wrote optimistically in *The Youngest Science*. Thomas presaged a time when all-knowing, high-precision instruments would measure and map all the functions of the human body, leaving little uncertainty and even fewer constraints or gaps in knowledge. "The new medicine works," he wrote. "The physician has the same obligations that he carried, overworked and often despairingly, fifty years ago—but now with any number of technological maneuvers to be undertaken quickly and with precision. . . . The hospitalized patient feels, for a time, like a working part of an immense, automated apparatus. He is admitted and discharged by batteries of computers, sometimes without even learning the doctors' names. Many patients go home speedily, in good health, cured of their diseases. . . . If I were a medical student or an intern, just getting ready to begin, I would be more worried about this aspect of my profession. I would be apprehensive that my real job, taking care of sick people, might soon be taken away, leaving me with the quite different occupation of looking after machines."

In reality, things have panned out quite differently: despite the increasing accuracy of tests, studies, and equipment, the doctors of today have to contend with priors, outliers, and biases with even deeper and more thoughtful engagement than doctors of the past. This is not a paradox. Tests and therapies may have evolved, but so has medicine itself. In Lewis Carroll's *Through the Looking-Glass*, the Red Queen tells a bewildered Alice that the queen has to keep running to stay in place—because the world keeps running in the opposite direction. Despite the sophistication of medical technologies, uncertainties have remained endemic to medicine because the projects that medicine has taken on are vastly more complex and ambitious. Thomas imagined a future in which machines took care of sick people. Now we have better machines, but we are using them to take care of sicker people.

In Philadelphia, a six-year-old girl with a lethal, therapy-resistant, relapsed leukemia recently had her immune cells harvested, genetically modified with a virus carrying a gene that kills leukemia cells, and then reinjected into her body to act as a form of "live" chemotherapy. The cells sought out and killed her cancer with exquisite efficacy, and she remains in a profound remission. At Emory, a neurosurgeon implanted a tiny electrical stimulator into the cingulate gyrus in the brain of a woman with profound depression. Seconds after the "brain pacemaker" was pulsed on, the woman described the lifting of a permanent dark fog of despair that had been recalcitrant to the highest doses of antidepressant medicines.

The Philadelphia experiment illustrates the nature of the complexities and uncertainties faced by the new medicine. Hours after the young girl with relapsed leukemia was injected with her cancer-seeking T cells, she experienced the most potent form of inflammatory response. Her physiology sensed the macabre aberration of her "self" turning on itself—an immune system attacking its own body (in fact, her T cells were attacking her cancer cells)—and she spiked a fever. Her blood pressure dropped. Her kidneys began to falter, her vessels began to clot and bleed at the same time, and she lapsed into a coma. A fleet of lab tests was sent out to monitor her status, and dozens returned with abnormal values. Which of these were the outliers, and which were the abnormal factors truly contributing to her terrifying inflammatory response? Her blood counts indicated that she might be in the beginnings of a remission—but was there an inherent bias in using these parameters to judge a remission in the setting of an acute inflammatory response?

Of all the abnormal lab values—every number capitalized, bolded, and flagged in violent red—one skyrocketing factor caught the eye of her physicians. Why? Because some prior knowledge indicated that the factor, called interleukin-6, or IL-6, sat at the hub of the inflammatory response. But also because there happened to be a drug against it: by pure chance, the leader of this trial happened to have a daughter who happened to have juvenile arthritis who happened to have been treated with a medication that blocked interleukin-6. Two days after the young girl's initial T-cell transfusion, doctors and nurses were pulling things off the shelves to see if any agent might work against the immune attack and consequent organ failure. "She was as sick as any human can possibly be," one physician recalled. Her vital signs fluttered on a precipice. In a last-ditch maneuver, she was injected with the antiarthritis drug. As the doctors watched, bewildered, the fever reversed. The kidneys, lungs, blood, and the heart returned to normal function. By the next morning, she awoke from her coma. One year later, she remains in remission, with no sign of cancer in her bone marrow.

Is the case over? Far from it. Should this girl be given chemotherapy now to "consolidate" her remission—as conventional wisdom might suggest—or would the added chemotherapy kill the very cells in her immune system that are keeping her disease in check? We don't know because there are no priors. Is her response normal, or is she an outlier? We won't know until we can build a model of the nature of her response and try to make all the available data fit it. How will we objectively judge this therapy in a clinical trial when no other comparable therapies for relapsed, refractory leukemia exist? Can such a trial ever be randomized?

This experiment—and hundreds of similar studies at the frontiers of medicine—suggest that human decision making, and, particularly, decision making in the face of uncertain, inaccurate, and imperfect information, remains absolutely vital to the life of medicine. There is no way around it. "The [political] revolution will not be tweeted," wrote Malcolm Gladwell. Well, the medical revolution will not be algorithmized.

....

One last thought: there is no reason to believe that there are only three laws of medicine. My own laws are personal. They stood by me throughout my internship, residency, and fellowship. They saved me from the most egregious errors of judgment; they helped me diagnose and treat the most difficult of the cases that I encountered in my practice. Every year, I begin my teaching rounds at the hospital by explaining my version of the laws to the new medical residents. Each time I see a new patient in the wards or in the clinic, I remind myself of them.

Yet if there are other laws, I suspect that they will also concern the nature of information and uncertainty at their very core. "Doctors," Voltaire wrote, "are men who prescribe medicines of which they know little, to cure diseases of which they know less, in human beings of whom they know nothing." The pivotal word in this scathing description is *know*. The discipline of medicine concerns the manipulation of knowledge under uncertainty. Abstract away the smell of rubbing alcohol and bleach; forget the adjustable beds and ward signs and the gleaming granite of hospital lobbies; erase, for a moment, the many corporeal indignities of a man in a blue cotton gown in a room or the doctor trying to heal him—and you have a discipline that is still learning to reconcile pure knowledge with real knowledge. The "youngest science" is also the most human science. It might well be the most beautiful and fragile thing that we do.

. . . .

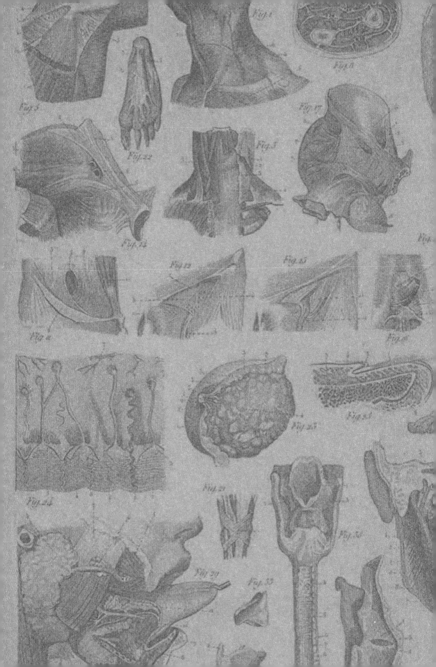

Fig. 5.
Fig. 22.
Fig. 1.
Fig. 8.
Fig. 17.
Fig. 3.
Fig. 14.
Fig. 18.
Fig. 12.
Fig. 15.
Fig. 11.
Fig. 19.
Fig. 25.
Fig. 23.
Fig. 24.
Fig. 28.
Fig. 21.
Fig. 26.
Fig. 20.
Fig. 33.

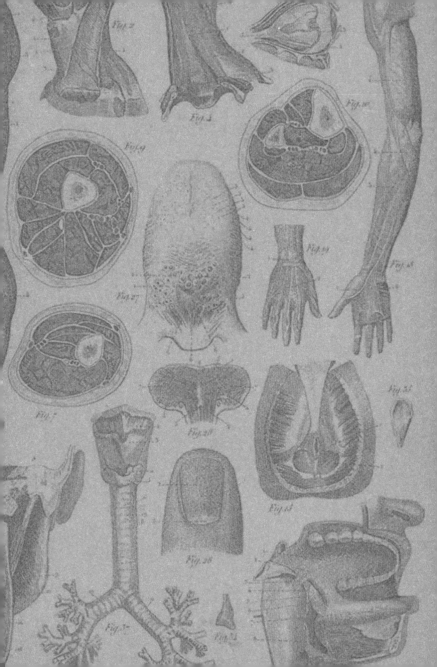

Siddhartha Mukherjee is a cancer physician and researcher. He is the author of *The Laws of Medicine* and *The Emperor of All Maladies: A Biography of Cancer*, winner of the 2011 Pulitzer Prize in general nonfiction. Mukherjee is an assistant professor of medicine at Columbia University and a staff cancer physician at Columbia University Medical Center. A Rhodes scholar, he graduated from Stanford University, University of Oxford, and Harvard Medical School. He has published articles in *Nature*, *Cell*, *The New England Journal of Medicine*, and *The New York Times*. In 2015, Mukherjee collaborated with Ken Burns on a six-hour, three-part PBS documentary on the history and future of cancer. Mukherjee's scientific work concerns cancer and stem cells, and his laboratory is known for the discovery of novel aspects of stem cell biology, including the isolation of stem cells that form bone and cartilage. He lives in New York with his wife and two daughters.

ACKNOWLEDGMENTS

I'd like to thank Michelle Quint for her careful editing of the manuscript and her remarkable equanimity in guiding this book to its final form. June Cohen and Chris Anderson helped shape a very shapeless idea of "laws" into this book. I owe a special debt to Sarah Sze, Nell Breyer, Sujoy Bhattacharyya, Suman Shirokar, Gerald Fischbach, Brittany Rush, and Ashok Rai for their comments and criticisms and to Bill Helman for helping me understand some of the most important ideas about uncertainty and the future of technology.

WATCH SIDDHARTHA MUKHERJEE'S TED TALK

Siddhartha Mukherjee's TED Talk, available for free at TED.com, is the companion to *The Laws of Medicine*.

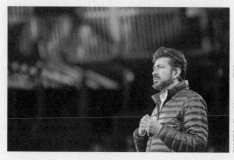

PHOTO: Bret Hartman/TED

RELATED TALKS ON TED.COM

Stefan Larsson
*What doctors can learn from
each other*
Different hospitals produce different
results on different procedures. Only
patients don't know that data, making
choosing a surgeon a high-stakes
guessing game. Stefan Larsson
looks at what happens when doctors
measure and share their outcomes on
hip replacement surgery, for example,
to see which techniques are proving
the most effective. Could health care
get better—and cheaper—if doctors
learn from each other in a continuous
feedback loop?

Abraham Verghese
A doctor's touch
Modern medicine is in danger of
losing a powerful, old-fashioned tool:
human touch. Physician and writer
Abraham Verghese describes our
strange new world where patients
are merely data points and calls for a
return to the traditional one-on-one
physical exam.

Atul Gawande
How do we heal medicine?
Our medical systems are broken.
Doctors are capable of extraordinary
(and expensive) treatments, but they
are losing their core focus: actually
treating people. Doctor and writer
Atul Gawande suggests we take a
step back and look at new ways to do
medicine—with fewer cowboys and
more pit crews.

Brian Goldman
*Doctors make mistakes. Can we talk
about that?*
Every doctor makes mistakes. But,
says physician Brian Goldman, medicine's culture of denial (and shame)
keeps doctors from ever talking about
those mistakes, or using them to learn
and improve. Telling stories from his
own long practice, he calls on doctors
to start talking about being wrong.

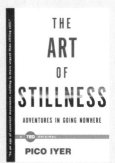

The Art of Stillness:
Adventures in Going Nowhere
by Pico Iyer

In a world beset by the distractions and demands of technology, acclaimed travel writer Pico Iyer reflects on why so many of us are desperate to unplug and bring stillness into our lives.

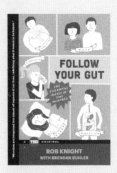

Follow Your Gut
The Enormous Impact of Tiny Microbes
by Rob Knight with Brendan Buhler

In this eye-opening book, scientist Rob Knight reveals how the microscopic life within our bodies—particularly within our intestines—has an astonishing impact on our lives. Your health, mood, sleep patterns, eating preferences, and more can all be traced in part to the tiny creatures that live on and inside of you.

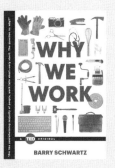

Why We Work
by Barry Schwartz

In this groundbreaking work, acclaimed writer and thinker Barry Schwartz dispels a deeply ingrained myth: The reason we work is primarily to get a paycheck. How did we come to believe this? Through fascinating studies and compelling anecdotes, Schwartz takes the reader on an eye-opening tour, illuminating the destructive way work operates in our culture and ultimately empowering readers to find their own path to good work.

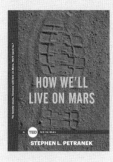

How We'll Live on Mars
by Stephen Petranek

Within 20 years, humans will live on Mars. We'll need to. Award-winning journalist Stephen Petranek makes the case that living on Mars is not just plausible, but inevitable, thanks to new technology and the competitive spirit of the world's most forward-looking entrepreneurs.

TED is a nonprofit devoted to spreading ideas, usually in the form of short, powerful talks (18 minutes or less). TED began in 1984 as a conference where Technology, Entertainment, and Design converged, and today covers almost all topics—from science to business to global issues—in more than 100 languages. Meanwhile, independently run TEDx events help share ideas in communities around the world.

TED is a global community, welcoming people from every discipline and culture who seek a deeper understanding of the world. We believe passionately in the power of ideas to change attitudes, lives, and, ultimately, the world. On TED .com, we're building a clearinghouse of free knowledge from the world's most inspired thinkers—and a community of curious souls to engage with ideas and each other, both online and at TED and TEDx events around the world, all year long.

In fact, everything we do—from our TED Talks videos to the projects sparked by the TED Prize, from the global TEDx community to the TED-Ed lesson series—is driven by this goal: How can we best spread great ideas?

TED is owned by a nonprofit, nonpartisan foundation.